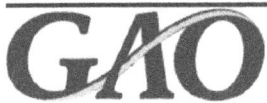

United States Government Accountability Office

Report to Congressional Requesters

May 2013

VA HEALTH CARE

Management and Oversight of Fee Basis Care Need Improvement

GAO-13-441

GAO Highlights

Highlights of GAO-13-441, a report to congressional requesters

May 2013

VA HEALTH CARE

Management and Oversight of Fee Basis Care Need Improvement

Why GAO Did This Study

While VA treats the majority of veterans in VA-operated facilities, in some instances it must obtain the services of non-VA providers to ensure that veterans are provided timely and accessible care. These non-VA providers are commonly reimbursed by VA using a fee-for-service arrangement known as fee basis care. VA's fee basis care program has grown rapidly in recent years—rising from about 8 percent of VA's total health care services budget in fiscal year 2005 to about 11 percent in fiscal year 2012. GAO was asked to review fee basis care program spending and utilization and factors that influence VAMC fee basis utilization. This report examines how fee basis care spending and utilization changed from fiscal year 2008 to fiscal year 2012, factors that contribute to the use of fee basis care, and VA's oversight of fee basis care program spending and utilization.

GAO reviewed relevant laws and regulations, VA policies, and fee basis spending and utilization data from fiscal year 2008 through fiscal year 2012. In addition, GAO reviewed the fee basis care operations of six selected VAMCs that varied in size, services offered, and geographic location.

What GAO Recommends

GAO recommends that VA revise its beneficiary travel regulations to allow reimbursement for veterans seeking similar care from a fee basis provider, apply the same wait time goals to fee basis care as VAMC-based care, and ensure fee basis data includes a claim number. VA generally concurred with GAO's conclusions and five recommendations.

View GAO-13-441. For more information, contact Randall Williamson at (202) 512-7114 or williamsonr@gao.gov.

What GAO Found

The Department of Veterans Affairs' (VA) fee basis care spending increased from about $3.04 billion in fiscal year 2008 to about $4.48 billion in fiscal year 2012. The slight decrease in fiscal year 2012 spending from the fiscal year 2011 level was due to VA's adoption of Medicare rates as its primary payment method for fee basis providers. VA's fee basis care utilization also increased from about 821,000 veterans in fiscal year 2008 to about 976,000 veterans in fiscal year 2012.

Total VA Fee Basis Care Spending, Fiscal Years 2008 through 2012

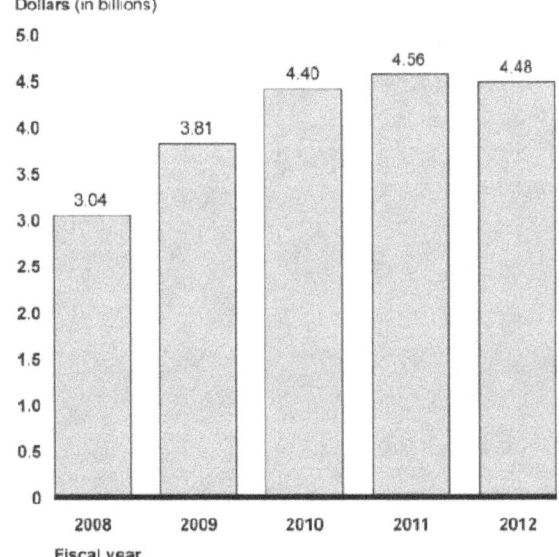

Source: GAO (analysis); VA (data).

GAO found that several factors affect VA medical centers' (VAMC) utilization of fee basis care—including veteran travel distances to VAMCs and goals for the maximum amount of time veterans should wait for VAMC-based appointments. VAMCs that GAO reviewed reported that they often use fee basis care to provide veterans with treatment closer to their homes—particularly for veterans who are not eligible for travel reimbursement. In addition, VAMC officials reported that veterans are often referred to fee basis providers to ensure that VAMC-based clinics that would otherwise treat them can meet established VA wait time goals for how long veterans wait for an appointment. However, GAO found that VA has not established goals for and does not track how long veterans wait to be seen by fee basis providers.

VA's monitoring of fee basis care spending is limited because fee basis data do not currently include a claim number or other identifier that allows all charges from a single office visit with a fee basis provider or an inpatient hospital stay to be analyzed together. GAO found that without the ability to analyze spending in this way, VA is limited in its ability to assess the cost of fee basis care and verify that fee basis providers were paid appropriately.

United States Government Accountability Office

Contents

Letter		1
	Background	4
	VA Fee Basis Care Spending and Utilization Increased from Fiscal Year 2008 to Fiscal Year 2012, with the Majority of Spending and Utilization in Outpatient Care	10
	Three Main Factors Influence Fee Basis Care Utilization, and VAMCs Reviewed Used Several Methods to Reduce Fee Basis Spending and Utilization	16
	VA's Processes for Overseeing the Fee Basis Care Program Lack Critical Data Needed to Effectively Track and Monitor Fee Basis Spending and Utilization	27
	VA Is Currently Implementing a Short-Term Corrective Action Plan for the Fee Basis Care Program, but Longer-Term Strategy Is Still in Development	30
	Conclusions	32
	Recommendations for Executive Action	33
	Agency Comments and Our Evaluation	34
Appendix I	VA Spending and Utilization by Fee Basis Care Category	38
Appendix II	VA Outpatient and Inpatient Spending and Utilization by Fee Basis Care Category	39
Appendix III	Comments from the Department of Veterans Affairs	41
Appendix IV	GAO Contact and Staff Acknowledgments	44

Tables

	Table 1: Status of Short-Term Improvement Goals, March 2013	31
	Table 2: VA Spending and Utilization by Fee Basis Care Category, Fiscal Years 2008 through 2012	38
	Table 3: Outpatient Spending and Utilization by VA Fee Basis Care Category, Fiscal Years 2008 through 2012	39

Table 4:	Inpatient Spending and Utilization by VA Fee Basis Care Category, Fiscal Years 2008 through 2012	40

Figures

Figure 1:	VA Medical Center (VAMC) Fee Basis Preauthorization Process Steps	5
Figure 2:	Veterans Integrated Service Network (VISN) or VA Medical Center (VAMC) Fee Basis Claims Processing Steps	7
Figure 3:	Veterans Health Administration (VHA) Chief Business Office (CBO) Oversight of Fee Basis Care	9
Figure 4:	Total VA Fee Basis Care Spending in Dollars, Fiscal Years 2008 through 2012	11
Figure 5:	Number of Unique Veterans Who Received Care from Fee Basis Providers, Fiscal Years 2008 through 2012	13
Figure 6:	VA Fee Basis Care Spending by Inpatient and Outpatient Care in Dollars, Fiscal Years 2008 through 2012	14
Figure 7:	Number of Unique Veterans Who Received Care from Inpatient and Outpatient Fee Basis Providers, Fiscal Years 2008 through 2012	15

Abbreviations

CBO	Chief Business Office
DOD	Department of Defense
HCPCS	Healthcare Common Procedure Coding System
MS-DRG	Medicare Severity Diagnosis Related Group
OIG	Office of Inspector General
VA	Department of Veterans Affairs
VAMC	VA medical center
VHA	Veterans Health Administration
VISN	Veterans Integrated Service Network

This is a work of the U.S. government and is not subject to copyright protection in the United States. The published product may be reproduced and distributed in its entirety without further permission from GAO. However, because this work may contain copyrighted images or other material, permission from the copyright holder may be necessary if you wish to reproduce this material separately.

GAO

U.S. GOVERNMENT ACCOUNTABILITY OFFICE

441 G St. N.W.
Washington, DC 20548

May 31, 2013

Congressional Requesters

The Department of Veterans Affairs (VA) treats the majority of eligible veterans it serves in VA-operated facilities, such as VA medical centers (VAMC).[1] However, in some instances, VA must obtain the services of non-VA providers to help ensure that veterans are provided timely and accessible care. These non-VA providers treat veterans in non-VA facilities, such as physicians' offices or hospitals in the community.[2] Non-VA providers are commonly paid by VA using a fee-for-service arrangement—known as fee basis care.[3] VA's fee basis care program has grown rapidly—in fiscal year 2005 VA's total spending on fee basis care was about $1.6 billion and represented about 8 percent of VA's total health care services budget, while in fiscal year 2012 VA's total spending on fee basis care was about $4.5 billion and represented about 11 percent of VA's total health care services budget.[4]

Although VA would prefer to deliver care to veterans within its own health care system operated by the Veterans Health Administration (VHA), officials recognize that it is necessary to use fee basis providers to help ensure that veterans are provided timely and accessible care.[5] For example, VA utilizes fee basis care when a VAMC is unable to provide certain specialty care services, such as cardiology or orthopedics, or

---

[1] VA's health care system includes 152 VAMCs. VA also provides care to veterans in VA-operated community-based outpatient clinics, community living centers (nursing homes), residential rehabilitation treatment programs, and comprehensive home care programs.

[2] VA obtains the services of non-VA providers in non-VA facilities under the following statutory authorities: 38 U.S.C. §§ 1703, 1725, 1728, 8111, and 8153. VA also has authority to employ providers on a fee basis to provide care in VA-operated facilities. See 38 U.S.C. § 7405(a)(2). This type of fee basis care is outside the scope of our report.

[3] While we refer to this program as fee basis care in this report, VA has renamed it non-VA medical care.

[4] These fee basis spending figures include all fee basis care for veterans provided by non-VA providers in non-VA facilities.

[5] Fee basis care can be delivered by different types of health care providers—including physicians, chiropractors, physical therapists, and psychologists. This care is often preapproved by the VAMC the veteran most frequently visits; however in certain circumstances, fee basis care can be used to provide emergency care to veterans.

when veterans must travel long distances to obtain specialty care from VA providers.

Congressional requesters have raised questions about the rising costs of fee basis care and issues with VA's management and oversight of its fee basis care program as highlighted in reports by the VA Office of Inspector General (OIG) and the National Academy of Public Administration.[6] These issues include a lack of internal controls for payment of fee basis providers and ineffective management and oversight of the fee basis care program by local and VA Central Office officials. VA has also acknowledged that while the fee basis program has seen marked growth in the number of veterans it serves, the management and support systems used to administer the program have not matured in a similar manner. In this report we examine: (1) how fee basis care spending and utilization have changed from fiscal year 2008 through fiscal year 2012; (2) factors that contribute to the use of fee basis care and steps some VAMCs are taking to reduce fee basis care; (3) VA's oversight of fee basis care program spending and utilization; and (4) VA's plans and strategies to improve the fee basis care program.

To examine how fee basis care spending and utilization have changed from fiscal year 2008 through fiscal year 2012, we reviewed fee basis data and interviewed officials from VA Central Office. Specifically, we reviewed four separate files of fee basis program data—inpatient records, inpatient ancillary records, outpatient records, and pharmacy-only records—for each fiscal year from 2008 through 2012. We analyzed these files separately and together to be able to report fee basis utilization and spending by fiscal year and across all 5 fiscal years.[7] We analyzed fee basis data for fiscal years 2008 through 2012 to determine: (1) the

---

[6]See Department of Veterans Affairs Office of Inspector General, *Audit of Veterans Health Administration's Non-VA Outpatient Fee Care Program*, 08-02901-185 (Washington D.C.: Aug. 3, 2009). This report found that in fiscal year 2008 VA made a significant number of improper payments—approximately 37 percent of paid claims. These improper payments included duplicate payments and payments processed for incorrect amounts. The VA OIG also concluded that VA needed to take immediate action to strengthen controls over the fee basis care program to ensure that payments were accurate and proper. See also National Academy of Public Administration, *Veterans Health Administration Fee Care Program* (Washington, D.C.: September 2011). This report was completed at VA's request and found that there were several challenges associated with the fee basis care program.

[7]In addition, we combined inpatient records and inpatient ancillary records together in order to conduct analyses on all inpatient data.

spending associated with inpatient and outpatient fee basis care, (2) how many veterans received inpatient and outpatient care from fee basis providers, and (3) the breakdown of fee basis care spending and utilization by fee basis category. Our final analysis of fee basis data included all records of fee basis care except those for pharmacy-only fee basis payments. We excluded pharmacy-only fee basis care because: it (1) represents a very small portion of fee basis care spending ($0.002 billion for fiscal years 2008 through 2012), (2) represents a very small portion of fee basis care utilization (11,750 unique veterans for fiscal years 2008 through 2012),[8] (3) applies only to reimbursements of veterans for medications that they paid for as part of emergency care that was reimbursed by VA, and (4) could not be separated out into service-connected and non-service-connected emergency care categories.[9] To ensure the reliability of these data, we interviewed VA Central Office officials responsible for maintaining and analyzing fee basis data and conducted automated checks of data fields to ensure that they contained complete information. Following these actions, we found information in this dataset to be sufficiently reliable for the purposes of this report.

To examine the factors that contribute to the use of fee basis care and the steps some VAMCs are taking to reduce fee basis care, we spoke with VAMC officials at selected VAMCs about the factors that influence fee basis care usage at these facilities and how officials at these facilities have reduced fee basis care spending and utilization. We selected six VAMCs that varied in terms of size, services offered, and geographic location, given that all VAMCs offer veterans fee basis care. These six VAMCs were located in Durham and Salisbury, North Carolina;

---

[8]Unique veterans refers to individual veterans treated by fee basis providers during the period of analysis.

[9]VA pays for emergency care provided by non-VA facilities under 38 U.S.C. § 1728 (emergency care generally for service-connected conditions) or 38 U.S.C. § 1725 (Veterans Millennium Health Care and Benefits Act emergency care for non-service-connected conditions). Separating fee basis care emergency spending under each of these separate authorities was a necessary component of our analysis. VA can also authorize and pay for emergency care provided by non-VA facilities under 38 U.S.C. § 1703. However, in our report emergency care paid for under this authority is accounted for under categories such as preauthorized inpatient and outpatient care rather than emergency care categories. Emergency care provided by fee basis providers is deemed preauthorized if the providers provide notification of a veteran's admission within 72 hours, and this care can be paid under 38 U.S.C. § 1703. VA does not categorize payments for emergency care made under 38 U.S.C. § 1703 separately from other types of fee basis care paid under this authority in its fee basis data.

Alexandria, Louisiana; Biloxi, Mississippi; Las Vegas, Nevada; and Loma Linda, California. We also spoke with officials in the three Veterans Integrated Service Networks (VISN) responsible for managing these six selected VAMCs.[10] Information obtained from these VISNs and VAMCs cannot be generalized to all VISNs and VAMCs. Finally, we reviewed relevant VA policies and procedures related to methods discussed by VAMC officials during these interviews.

To examine VA's oversight of fee basis care program spending and utilization, we spoke with VA Central Office staff responsible for monitoring the program. In addition, we assessed the content and structure of VA Central Office databases used to monitor the fee basis care program.

To examine VA's plans and strategies to improve the fee basis care program, we spoke with VA Central Office staff responsible for developing planned improvements. We also reviewed documentation of these planned improvements.

We conducted our performance audit from September 2012 to May 2013 in accordance with generally accepted government auditing standards. Those standards require that we plan and perform the audit to obtain sufficient, appropriate evidence to provide a reasonable basis for our findings and conclusions based on our audit objectives. We believe that the evidence obtained provides a reasonable basis for our findings and conclusions based on our audit objectives.

Background

Fee Basis Care Authorization Process

The two main fee basis care delivery methods—preauthorized care and emergency care—are approved using two different processes.[11] Preauthorizing fee basis care involves a multistep process conducted by

---

[10]VISNs oversee the day-to-day functions of VAMCs that are within their network. Each VAMC is assigned to a single VISN.

[11]Preauthorized fee basis care comprises the majority, about 60 percent, of fee basis care.

the VAMC that regularly serves a veteran.[12] The preauthorization process is initiated by a VA provider who submits a request for fee basis care to the VAMC's fee basis care unit, which is an administrative department within each VAMC that processes VA providers' fee basis care requests and verifies that fee basis care is necessary.[13] Once approved by the VAMC Chief of Staff or his or her designee, the veteran is notified of the approval and can choose any fee basis provider willing to accept VA payment at predetermined rates.[14] (See fig. 1.)

Figure 1: VA Medical Center (VAMC) Fee Basis Preauthorization Process Steps

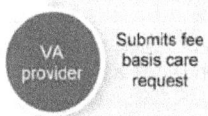 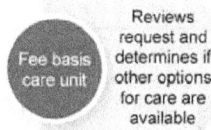 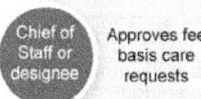 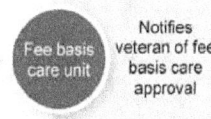 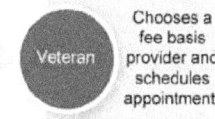

Source: GAO.

[a]In some VAMCs, the fee basis care unit may assist veterans in setting up their appointments with the fee basis provider of their choice.

In addition to preauthorizing fee basis care, VA also pays for fee basis care in certain emergency situations. For veterans with service-connected conditions, VA is required to pay for emergency care provided by non-VA facilities for service-connected conditions, medical conditions associated with or aggravating a service-connected condition, or for any condition if VA classifies the veteran as permanently and totally disabled due to their

---

[12]VA uses this same preauthorization process for nonemergency inpatient and outpatient care, dental care, nursing home care, compensation and pension exams, and most pharmacy expenses paid for through the fee basis care program.

[13]Most inpatient, outpatient, nursing home, dental, and pharmacy services provided through the fee basis care program are preauthorized.

[14]VA uses this process to preauthorize fee basis care from a number of different types of fee basis providers, including community-based hospitals and Department of Defense (DOD) medical facilities that collaborate with VAMCs to provide some veterans' care.

service-connected condition.[15] For veterans without service-connected conditions, VA must pay for emergency fee basis care if the veteran is enrolled in the VA healthcare system and has received VA care within the last 2 years, has no other health coverage, and satisfies certain other requirements.[16,17]

Fee Basis Care Payment Process

Regardless of whether a veteran's fee basis care was preauthorized or the result of an emergency, the steps for processing payments to fee basis providers are the same. Specifically, the fee basis provider submits a bill with a list of charges—commonly referred to as a claim—to either the VISN or VAMC for payment following the veteran's treatment. In some VISNs, claims processing activities are centralized in a VISN-level fee

---

[15] Under 38 U.S.C. § 1728, VA is required to pay for emergency care provided by non-VA facilities for service-connected conditions, non-service-connected conditions associated with and aggravating a service-connected condition, any condition if VA classifies the veteran as permanently and totally disabled due to a service-connected condition, and any condition for veterans participating in a vocational rehabilitation program who need care to participate in a course of training.

[16] Under 38 U.S.C. § 1725, as added by the 1999 Veterans Millennium Health Care and Benefits Act, VA is required to pay for emergency care provided by non-VA facilities for certain veterans that are not eligible for non-VA emergency care under section 1728. In order for a veteran's non-service-connected emergency conditions to be covered, veterans must be personally liable for the emergency care and must be active VA health care participants. To be an active VA health care participant, a veteran must be enrolled in the VA health care system and must have received VA care within the 2 years prior to receiving the emergency care. To be personally liable, a veteran must (1) be financially liable for the emergency care he or she receives; (2) have no entitlement or health care coverage under another health plan, such as Medicare or private health insurance; (3) have no other contractual or legal recourse against a third party that would in whole extinguish liability to the emergency care provider, such as insurance claims for car accidents; and (4) not be eligible under section 1728. The emergency care provided must be in response to a medical emergency, be provided when a VA or other federal facility was not feasibly available to provide the emergency care, and is limited to the services needed until transfer to a VA facility could be arranged. In addition, VA's regulations under the statute provide that the veteran must be treated in a hospital emergency department or similar facility; and the provider or the veteran must file a claim with VA within 90 days of providing the veteran's treatment, date of death, or the date the veteran exhausted, without success, action to obtain third-party payment. See 38 C.F.R. §§ 17.1000-17.1008.

[17] VA can also authorize and pay for emergency care provided by non-VA facilities under 38 U.S.C § 1703. However, in our report emergency care paid for under this authority is accounted for under categories such as preauthorized inpatient and outpatient care rather than emergency care categories. Emergency care provided by fee basis providers is deemed preauthorized if the providers provide notification of a veteran's admission within 72 hours, and this care can be paid under 38 U.S.C. § 1703. VA does not categorize payments for emergency care made under 38 U.S.C. § 1703 separately from other types of fee basis care paid under this authority in its fee basis data.

basis claims processing unit that is responsible for reviewing fee basis provider claims, obtaining copies of medical records for veterans' fee basis care, and approving payment to fee basis providers. In other VISNs, these claims-processing activities are decentralized and are the responsibility of individual VAMCs. After VAMC or VISN officials review the claims for accuracy, fee basis providers are reimbursed by VA. (See fig. 2.)

Figure 2: Veterans Integrated Service Network (VISN) or VA Medical Center (VAMC) Fee Basis Claims Processing Steps

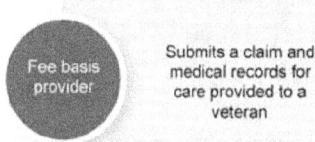
Fee basis provider — Submits a claim and medical records for care provided to a veteran

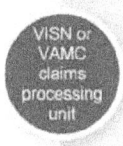
VISN or VAMC claims processing unit — Reviews claim for accuracy, determines reimbursement rate, and authorizes payment

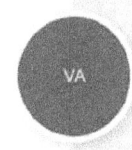
VA — Reimburses fee basis provider

Source: GAO.

Fee Basis Payment Rates

Prior to 2011, VA paid fee basis providers' claims using its own internally developed fee schedule or other local agreements.[18] In February 2011, VA began using applicable Medicare rates as its basis for reimbursing fee basis providers for all inpatient and outpatient services.[19] Medicare rates are generally lower than rates VA previously used to reimburse fee basis

---

[18] According to VA officials, prior to 2011, some VISNs and VAMCs had agreements with fee basis providers to pay claims at either applicable Medicare rates or other negotiated rates and fee basis hospital services were already paid at rates similar to Medicare rates. See 38 C.F.R. § 17.55.

[19] See 75 Fed. Reg. 78.901 (Dec. 17, 2010) (amending 38 C.F.R. §§ 17.52, 17.56). In December 2010, VA amended its regulations to apply Medicare rates, set by the Centers for Medicare & Medicaid Services, to all inpatient and outpatient care delivered by fee basis providers under 38 U.S.C. § 1703 and 38 U.S.C. § 1728. Emergency treatment provided under 38 U.S.C. § 1725 (Millennium Act) is reimbursed according to 38 C.F.R. § 17.1005, which specifies that reimbursement for care provided under the Millennium Act is reimbursed at the lesser of two payment options: (1) the amount for which the veteran is personally liable or (2) 70 percent of the amount specified in the applicable Medicare fee schedule for such treatment.

providers.[20] However, with the move to Medicare rates, some fee basis claims are paid at non-Medicare rates; specifically, if VA has a sharing or negotiated agreement with a fee basis provider that includes a non-Medicare rate, VA will pay that amount instead of the Medicare rate.[21] These rates are specific to each individual agreement and can be higher or lower than the Medicare rate. For example, some VAMCs currently provide dialysis treatments to veterans through preauthorized fee basis care using a multi-VISN negotiated rate that exceeds the Medicare reimbursement rate. Some VAMCs pay these higher reimbursement rates for fee basis dialysis care because the major fee basis dialysis providers did not agree to provide dialysis treatment to veterans at the Medicare reimbursement rate. In addition, many sharing agreements between VAMCs and DOD medical facilities allow VA to reimburse DOD for care it provides to veterans at a lower rate than Medicare.

VA Oversight of Fee Basis Care

VA Central Office has primary responsibility for overseeing VISNs' and VAMCs' fee basis care operations and manages the fee basis care program through the Veterans Health Administration (VHA) Chief Business Office (CBO).[22] According to VHA CBO officials, VHA CBO relies on three main methods for overseeing fee basis spending and utilization:

- **Reports from VISNs and VAMCs.** VISNs and VAMCs submit monthly reports that include information on their progress meeting several performance measures related to claims processing—including the total number of claims processed by each fee basis unit, the number of claims processed in 30 days or less, the number of claims processed in more than 30 days, and the number of appeals for payment of denied fee basis claims submitted by veterans.[23]

---

[20]Medicare pays for services such as those provided by physicians, inpatient hospitals, and dialysis facilities based on predetermined rates that are adjusted based on provider characteristics, geographical differences in market conditions, and other factors.

[21]See 38 C.F.R. § 17.56(a)(1).

[22]Within VA, VHA is the organization responsible for providing health care to veterans at medical facilities across the country.

[23]According to VHA CBO officials, VA Central Office set a goal for all VISN and VAMC fee basis units to process fee basis provider claims within 30 days of receipt.

- **Management reviews of VISN and VAMC operations.** VHA CBO staff conduct periodic site visits to examine a VISN or VAMC fee basis unit's claims processing functions and program monitoring to identify areas where the facility could improve. At the conclusion of these site visits, the VHA CBO staff that conducted the site visit prepares a formal report on the findings of the visit, including recommendations to improve processes, and provides training to the facility if needed.

- **Analysis of fee basis data.** VHA CBO staff regularly analyze fee basis claims data to gain a system-wide view of the fee basis care program. Specifically, they conduct retroactive reviews of fee basis data to identify cases of fraud, waste, and abuse; provide updates to VA stakeholders, including other key officials within VA Central Office, on the status of the fee basis care program; and independently verify findings from external reviews, including VA OIG audits.

According to VHA CBO officials, the Program Oversight and Informatics division is responsible for analyzing fee basis data to review overall trends and identify outliers in payments made to fee basis providers and the Program Administration division is responsible for conducting periodic reviews of VISN and VAMC fee basis operations and reviewing reports from VISNs and VAMCs on fee basis utilization. (See fig. 3.)

Figure 3: Veterans Health Administration (VHA) Chief Business Office (CBO) Oversight of Fee Basis Care

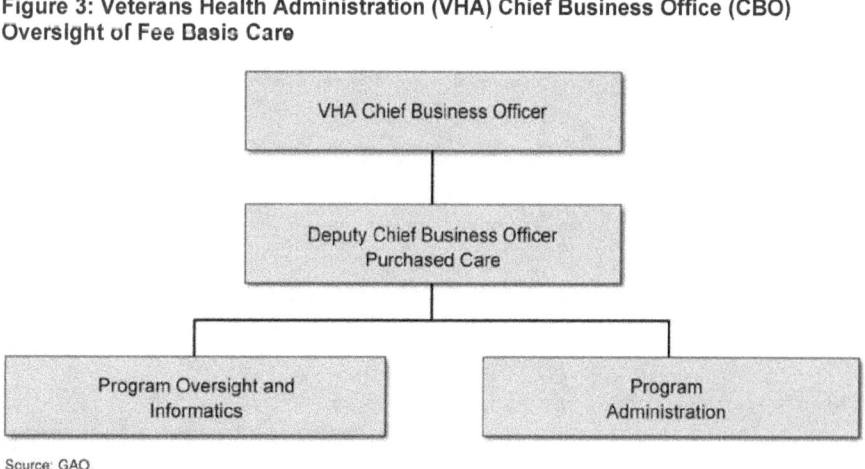

Source: GAO.

VA Fee Basis Care Spending and Utilization Increased from Fiscal Year 2008 to Fiscal Year 2012, with the Majority of Spending and Utilization in Outpatient Care

VA Fee Basis Care Spending and Utilization Increased from Fiscal Year 2008 to Fiscal Year 2012

VA's fee basis care spending increased from about $3.04 billion in fiscal year 2008 to about $4.48 billion in fiscal year 2012.[24] VA's fee basis care spending hit its highest level of about $4.56 billion in fiscal year 2011. Across the 5 fiscal years we reviewed, VA spent a total of about $20.29 billion on fee basis care. (See fig. 4.)

---

[24]Fee basis spending in this report does not include pharmacy-only fee basis care. Pharmacy-only fee basis care consists of reimbursements to veterans for medications that they paid for as part of emergency care that was reimbursed by VA under 38 U.S.C. § 1728 (emergency care generally for service-connected conditions) or 38 U.S.C. § 1725 (Veterans Millennium Health Care and Benefits Act emergency care for non-service-connected conditions). Total spending for pharmacy-only fee basis care was $0.002 billion for fiscal years 2008 through 2012.

Figure 4: Total VA Fee Basis Care Spending in Dollars, Fiscal Years 2008 through 2012

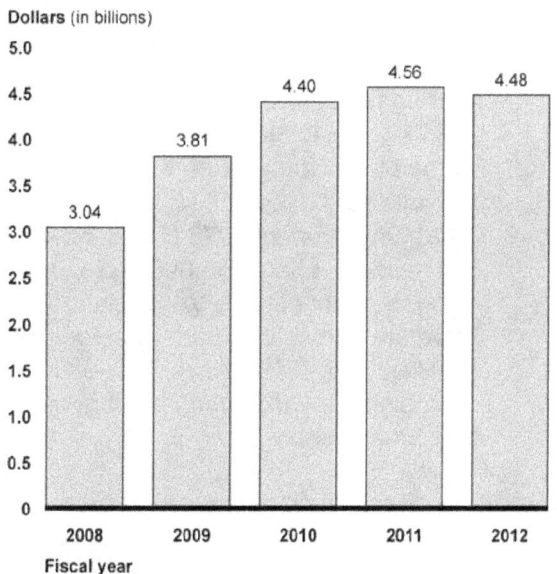

Source: GAO (analysis); VA (data).

Notes: Fee basis spending in this figure does not include pharmacy-only fee basis care. Pharmacy-only fee basis care consists of reimbursements to veterans for medications that they paid for as part of emergency care that was reimbursed by VA under 38 U.S.C. § 1728 (emergency care generally for service-connected conditions) or 38 U.S.C. § 1725 (Veterans Millennium Health Care and Benefits Act emergency care for non-service-connected conditions). Total spending for pharmacy-only fee basis care was $0.002 billion for fiscal years 2008 through 2012.

Spending totals in this figure have been rounded.

The overall increase in fee basis care spending from fiscal year 2008 to fiscal year 2012 can be attributed to increases in the number of veterans who received fee basis care. The slight decline in fee basis care spending between fiscal year 2011 and fiscal year 2012 is likely due to VA's adoption of Medicare rates for its fee basis care program. Medicare reimbursement rates are typically lower for most health care services than VA's previous fee basis care reimbursement rates.[25]

VA's fee basis care utilization also increased from fiscal year 2008 to fiscal year 2012—although the number of unique veterans receiving care from fee basis providers has increased less rapidly for the last 3 fiscal years.[26] A total of about 2.45 million unique veterans received care from fee basis providers from fiscal year 2008 to fiscal year 2012.[27] Total fee basis care utilization hit its highest point of the 5-year period in fiscal year 2012 when about 976,000 unique veterans received care from fee basis providers, about 155,000 more veterans than in fiscal year 2008. (See fig. 5.) According to VA officials, the increase in the number of unique veterans receiving care from fee basis providers from fiscal year 2008 to fiscal year 2012 was likely due to VA's use of fee basis care to meet goals for the maximum amount of time veterans wait for VAMC-based appointments.

---

[25] See GAO, *VA Health Care: Methodology for Estimating and Process for Tracking Savings Need Improvement*, GAO-12-305 (Washington, D.C.: Feb. 27, 2012). VA began using Medicare reimbursement rates for its fee basis program in February 2011. By reimbursing fee basis providers at the Medicare rate for the care they provide veterans, VA estimated that it would be able to save $315 million in fiscal year 2012 and $362 million in fiscal year 2013. In addition, some savings would have been achieved during fiscal year 2011 as a result of these rates being used for 7 months of fiscal year 2011.

[26] Fee basis utilization in this report does not include pharmacy-only fee basis care. Pharmacy-only fee basis care consists of reimbursements to veterans for medications that they paid for as part of emergency care that was reimbursed by VA under 38 U.S.C. § 1728 (emergency care generally for service-connected conditions) or 38 U.S.C. § 1725 (Veterans Millennium Health Care and Benefits Act emergency care for non-service-connected conditions). A total of 11,750 unique veterans received such reimbursement from fiscal year 2008 through fiscal year 2012.

[27] Unique veterans refers to individual veterans treated during the period of analysis and ensures that the number of veterans served by the fee basis care program is not overstated due to some veterans being treated by fee basis providers more than once. To determine the total number of unique veterans who received care from fee basis providers (about 2.45 million), we counted each individual veteran only once for the 5-year period by identifying the number of unique Social Security numbers present in fee basis data.

Figure 5: Number of Unique Veterans Who Received Care from Fee Basis Providers, Fiscal Years 2008 through 2012

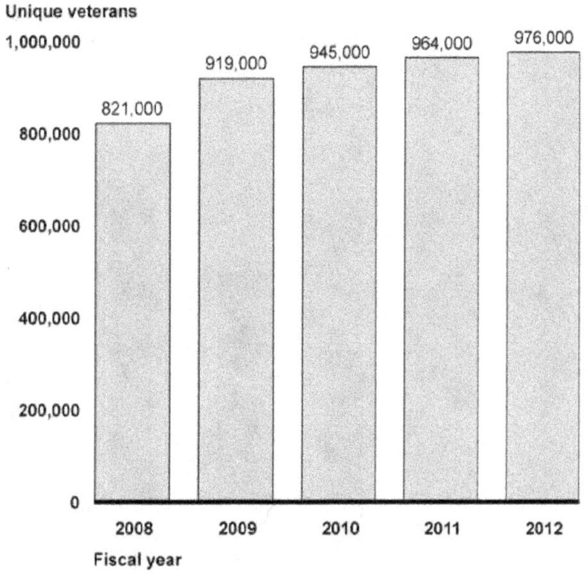

Unique veterans

Fiscal year	Unique veterans
2008	821,000
2009	919,000
2010	945,000
2011	964,000
2012	976,000

Source: GAO (analysis); VA (data).

Notes: Fee basis utilization in this figure does not include pharmacy-only fee basis care. Pharmacy-only fee basis care consists of reimbursements to veterans for medications that they paid for as part of emergency care that was reimbursed by VA under 38 U.S.C. § 1728 (emergency care generally for service-connected conditions) or 38 U.S.C. § 1725 (Veterans Millennium Health Care and Benefits Act emergency care for non-service-connected conditions). A total of 11,750 unique veterans received such reimbursement from fiscal year 2008 through fiscal year 2012.

To determine the fee basis utilization numbers in this figure, we counted each individual veteran once per fiscal year by identifying the number of unique Social Security numbers present in each fiscal year's fee basis data. Utilization totals in this figure have been rounded to the nearest thousand veterans.

In addition, fee basis care spending and utilization also varied by fee basis care category. (See app. I for more information.)

Outpatient Services Accounted for the Majority of VA Fee Basis Care Spending and Utilization from Fiscal Year 2008 through Fiscal Year 2012

VA spent about $11.22 billion on outpatient fee basis care and about $9.07 billion on inpatient fee basis care from fiscal year 2008 through fiscal year 2012. During this 5-year period, inpatient fee basis care spending increased steadily from about $1.41 billion in fiscal year 2008 to about $2.15 billion in fiscal year 2012, while outpatient fee basis care spending declined in fiscal year 2012. As a result, by fiscal year 2012, the difference in inpatient and outpatient fee basis care spending was only about $180 million, compared to a $590 million disparity in fiscal year

2011 when outpatient fee basis care spending was at its highest level. (See fig. 6.)

Figure 6: VA Fee Basis Care Spending by Inpatient and Outpatient Care in Dollars, Fiscal Years 2008 through 2012

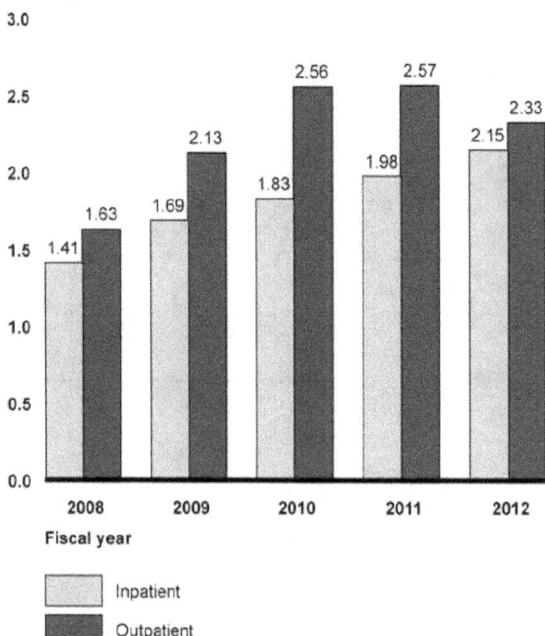

Source: GAO (analysis); VA (data).

Notes: Fee basis spending in this figure does not include pharmacy-only fee basis care. Pharmacy-only fee basis care consists of reimbursements to veterans for medications that they paid for as part of emergency care that was reimbursed by VA under 38 U.S.C. § 1728 (emergency care generally for service-connected conditions) or 38 U.S.C. § 1725 (Veterans Millennium Health Care and Benefits Act emergency care for non-service-connected conditions). Total spending for pharmacy-only fee basis care was $0.002 billion for fiscal years 2008 through 2012.

Spending totals in this figure have been rounded.

Significantly more veterans received care from outpatient fee basis care providers than from inpatient fee basis care providers. Specifically, from fiscal year 2008 through fiscal year 2012, a total of about 2.35 million unique veterans received care from outpatient fee basis providers and a total of about 472,000 unique veterans received care from inpatient fee basis providers.[28] (See fig. 7.)

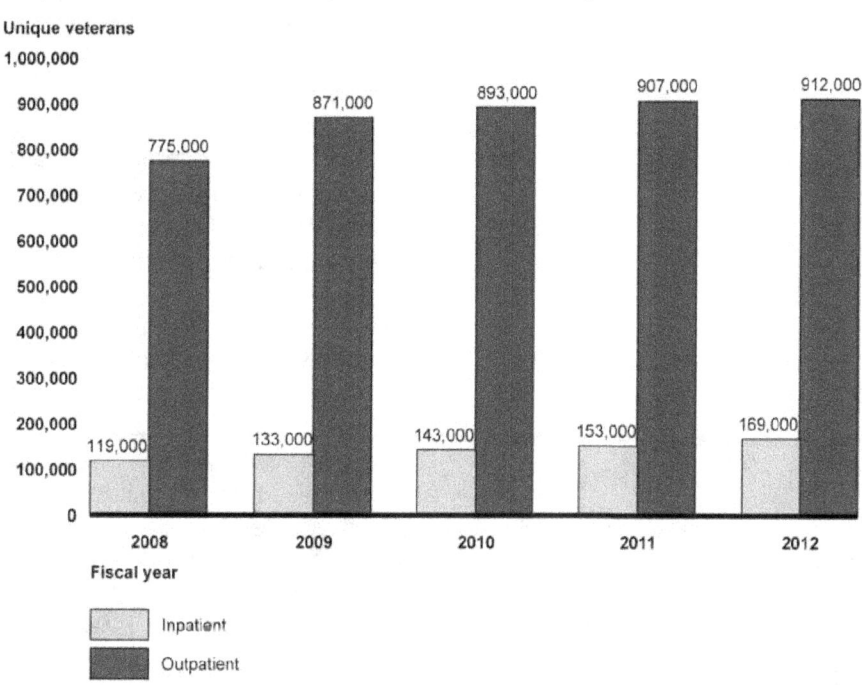

Figure 7: Number of Unique Veterans Who Received Care from Inpatient and Outpatient Fee Basis Providers, Fiscal Years 2008 through 2012

Source: GAO (analysis); VA (data).

Notes: Fee basis utilization in this figure does not include pharmacy-only fee basis care. Pharmacy-only fee basis care consists of reimbursements to veterans for medications that they paid for as part of emergency care that was reimbursed by VA under 38 U.S.C. § 1728 (emergency care generally for service-connected conditions) or 38 U.S.C. § 1725 (Veterans Millennium Health Care and Benefits Act emergency care for non-service-connected conditions). A total of 11,750 unique veterans received such reimbursement from fiscal year 2008 through fiscal year 2012.

Utilization amounts in this figure may not match utilization totals cited previously in text, as some veterans may have received both inpatient and outpatient fee basis care during the same fiscal year. To determine the inpatient fee basis utilization numbers in this figure, we counted each individual

---

[28] To determine the number of unique veterans who received care from outpatient fee basis providers (2.35 million), we counted each individual veteran only once for the 5-year period by identifying the number of unique Social Security numbers present in outpatient fee basis data. To determine the number of unique veterans who received care from inpatient fee basis providers (472,000), we counted each individual veteran only once for the 5-year period by identifying the number of unique Social Security numbers present in inpatient fee basis data. These fee basis utilization figures have been rounded.

veteran once per fiscal year by identifying the number of unique Social Security numbers present in inpatient fee basis data. To determine the outpatient fee basis utilization numbers in this figure, we counted each individual veteran once per fiscal year by identifying the number or unique Social Security numbers present in outpatient fee basis data. These fee basis utilization totals have been rounded.

Preauthorized fee basis care accounted for the majority of outpatient fee basis spending and utilization from fiscal year 2008 through fiscal year 2012—about $7.36 billion and about 80 percent of unique veterans receiving outpatient fee basis care. VA spent the least on outpatient fee basis care for compensation and pension exams and emergency care for service-connected veterans.[29] In addition, preauthorized fee basis care accounted for the majority of inpatient fee basis care spending from fiscal year 2008 through fiscal year 2012. Preauthorized inpatient fee basis care accounted for about $4.60 billion and about 57 percent of unique veterans receiving inpatient fee basis care. VA spent the least on inpatient fee basis care associated with emergency care for service-connected veterans. (See App. II.)

Three Main Factors Influence Fee Basis Care Utilization, and VAMCs Reviewed Used Several Methods to Reduce Fee Basis Spending and Utilization

During our review of six VAMCs, we identified three common factors that affected these facilities' utilization of fee basis care—clinical service availability, veteran travel distances, and VA wait time goals. In addition, officials from the six VAMCs reported several methods they use to reduce either the cost of referring veterans to fee basis providers or the number of veterans their facilities refer to fee basis providers.

---

[29]Emergency care for service-connected veterans refers to fee basis care that meets the eligibility requirements for emergency care under 38 U.S.C. § 1728. Under this statute, VA is required to pay for emergency care provided by non-VA facilities for service-connected conditions, non-service-connected conditions associated with and aggravating a service-connected condition, any condition if the veteran is classified by VA as permanently and totally disabled from a service-connected condition, and any condition for veterans participating in a vocational rehabilitation program who need care to participate in a course of training.

Limited Availability of Clinical Services, Veteran Travel Distances, and Wait Times Goals Influence Fee Basis Care Utilization

Limited Availability of Clinical Services

VAMCs have limitations on the services they can offer due to a variety of factors, including the size of their facilities and the types of providers they can recruit, which can affect fee basis care utilization. VA officials from the six VAMCs we examined reported that the types of clinical services offered at their facilities affected veterans' utilization of fee basis care. For example, officials from the Alexandria VAMC explained that their facility does not meet VA's requirements for providing orthopedic surgery services to veterans and does not provide these services. As a result, they refer veterans who need these services to fee basis providers. Similarly, officials from the Biloxi VAMC explained that they do not have the ability to offer radiation therapy for cancer treatment at their medical center. As a result, they refer veterans who need radiation therapy to fee basis providers and reported that their VAMC has little control over increases in fee basis spending for these services.

In some cases, a VAMC may not be able to provide some services to veterans because they do not have the right mix of clinical specialists to accommodate complications that may arise during surgery. For example, for a VAMC to offer joint replacement surgery, the facility must be equipped with an orthopedic specialist capable of performing the surgery and a number of additional providers to assist in the event of an emergency complication during surgery. For joint replacement surgeries, these additional providers include a thoracic surgeon and a neurologist who both must be available within 15 minutes by phone or 60 minutes in person, if needed. If these criteria for additional providers are not met, the VAMC is not authorized to perform joint replacement surgeries even if the VAMC has an orthopedic specialist capable of performing the surgery. When VAMCs are unable to provide services due to these requirements, they may rely on fee basis care to obtain these services for veterans.

In other cases, VAMCs are unable to recruit specialists and as a result cannot offer some clinical services to veterans. When such recruiting challenges arise, VAMCs may rely on fee basis care to ensure veterans can receive medical services. For example, officials from the Las Vegas VAMC explained that they have difficulty recruiting several types of specialists—including vascular surgeons, pulmonologists, and gastroenterologists. These officials explained that they are exploring ways to provide relocation incentives to help recruit specialists; however, they noted recruiting is difficult because recent medical school graduates often want the opportunity to conduct medical research in addition to patient care and the Las Vegas VAMC does not have a research program.

Veteran Travel Distances to VAMCs

The distance that veterans have to travel to receive medical care is also a critical factor influencing whether they are treated in VAMCs or referred to fee basis providers. Traveling long distances for medical care is often impractical for veterans, particularly those receiving ongoing outpatient medical care, such as dialysis or radiation therapy for cancer. The decision about whether a veteran can physically tolerate the travel to a VAMC or should be referred to a fee basis provider in the community is a clinical judgment VA providers make in consultation with VAMC fee basis care unit staff. Officials from all six of the VAMCs we reviewed reported that utilization of fee basis care was affected by the distance that veterans must travel to receive VAMC-based care. For example, the Biloxi VAMC serves veterans from four states along the Gulf Coast, including many who live more than 300 miles from the facility. Officials from the Biloxi VAMC explained that the significant travel distance that some veterans face when traveling from their homes to the VAMC for care is burdensome and may not be appropriate for all veterans. As a result, these officials said that their VAMC frequently refers veterans to fee basis providers within the veterans' own communities to reduce this burden. Similarly, officials from the Alexandria VAMC explained that many times they also refer veterans to fee basis providers in veterans' own communities to lessen the travel burden.

Another related factor that can increase fee basis utilization involves whether veterans referred to fee basis providers are eligible for reimbursement for travel costs through VA's beneficiary travel program. VA's beneficiary travel program reimburses eligible veterans for travel from their home to either their primary VAMC, another VAMC, or to a fee basis provider that can provide the care they need.[30] Under VA's beneficiary travel program regulations, veterans are eligible for travel reimbursement only if they meet one of several criteria—including having

---

[30]See Veterans Health Administration, *Beneficiary Travel*, Handbook 1601B.05 (July 23, 2010). Through VA's beneficiary travel program eligible veterans may receive reimbursement for travel expenses for any distance if it is financially favorable to the government.

a service-connected disability rating of 30 percent or more, or an annual income below a specified threshold.[31] Therefore, veterans who do not meet these criteria cannot receive reimbursement for travel costs to another VAMC for treatment. Under these circumstances, veterans may see a fee basis provider closer to their residences, according to VA officials, even though fee basis care may cost VA considerably more than the cost of treatment in a VAMC. The Secretary of Veterans Affairs has authority under the beneficiary travel authorizing statute to provide travel reimbursement to additional categories of veterans. However, VAMCs only have the authority to reimburse veterans who meet the eligibility requirements of the beneficiary travel program as outlined in VA regulations.[32] In order to allow VAMCs to reimburse additional veterans for travel, VA would need to revise its regulations to include additional categories of veterans.

Officials from one VAMC and a few VISNs we reviewed told us they often send veterans who are not eligible for travel reimbursement to fee basis providers instead of referring them to other VAMCs that can provide the care because VA cannot compensate them for their travel to another VA facility. For example, officials from the Biloxi VAMC explained that the Houston VAMC is able to provide veterans with high-quality interventional cardiology services, such as cardiac catheterization and cardiothoracic

---

[31]Under 38 U.S.C. § 111, VA is authorized but not required to pay travel expenses for veterans. However, if VA exercises its authority to reimburse travel expenses, VA must pay travel expenses for specified categories of veterans and may reimburse travel expenses for any other veterans receiving medical care. Currently, VA's regulations for the beneficiary travel program designate as eligible the categories of veterans specifically mentioned in 38 U.S.C. § 111. See 38 C.F.R. § 70.10. Specifically, veterans must meet at least one of the following criteria: (1) have a service-connected disability rating of 30 percent or more; (2) be receiving care related to their service-connected disability if their service-connected disability rating is less than 30 percent; (3) be receiving VA pension benefits; (4) have an annual income below the maximum applicable annual rate of pension for all conditions ($12,465 for a veteran with no dependents in fiscal year 2013); (5) present clear evidence that they are unable to defray the cost of travel; or (6) be traveling to receive an exam to qualify them for VA compensation and pension. Veterans traveling for certain emergency situations may be eligible for transportation expenses under separate authority. See 38 U.S.C. § 1725; 38 C.F.R. §§ 17.1000–17.1008. Persons specifically mentioned in other VA statutes as eligible for payment for beneficiary travel are also eligible, such as certain family members of veterans. See 38 C.F.R. § 70.10. Not all veterans eligible for fee basis care are eligible for beneficiary travel benefits at VA.

[32]Currently, VA's beneficiary travel regulations limit eligibility for beneficiary travel to only those categories of veterans specifically mentioned in the beneficiary travel statute. See 38 U.S.C. § 111; 38 C.F.R. § 70.10.

surgery, which are not available at the Biloxi VAMC. However, if a veteran is not eligible for beneficiary travel, the Biloxi VAMC will refer them to a fee basis provider to lessen the financial burden on the veteran even though, in some cases, care from a fee basis provider may cost the Biloxi VAMC $30,000 to $40,000 more than if the veteran were treated at the Houston VAMC. Biloxi VAMC officials said that they have asked their VISN to allow them to reimburse additional veterans for travel to the Houston VAMC for services that facility can provide, but they were informed that VA's beneficiary travel regulations do not permit them to offer travel reimbursements to veterans not eligible for beneficiary travel benefits.

As part of the fee basis preauthorization process, VAMC or VISN officials do not evaluate whether it would be less expensive to send veterans to another VAMC for treatment rather than sending them to a fee basis provider. In requesting authorization for a veteran to see a fee basis provider, VAMC providers do not currently include information on the likely costs of the fee basis care.[33]

VA Wait Time Goals

The amount of time veterans wait for VAMC-based appointments for health care also may be a significant factor that increases VA's utilization of fee basis care. In fiscal year 2012, VA performance goals for VAMC-based care wait times called for VAMCs to complete veterans' primary care appointments within 7 days of their desired appointment date and schedule veterans' specialty care appointments within 14 days of their desired appointment date.[34] These performance goals are included in VISN and VAMC directors' annual performance contracts and are a part of the scores used to determine the amount of performance pay they are

---

[33] VA does require VA providers referring a veteran to a fee basis provider to enter one of five preprogrammed justifications in the request for fee basis care. These justifications include: (1) the VA facility does not provide the required service, (2) the veteran cannot safely travel to a VA facility due to a medical reason which must be specified, (3) the veteran cannot travel to a VA facility due to geographical inaccessibility, (4) the VA facility cannot provide the required service in a timely manner, or (5) "other" reasons, which must be specified. VA fee basis care units processing these referrals will not approve the veteran's fee basis care without one of these justifications from the VA provider.

[34] VA's policy for determining the desired appointment date is unclear. A veteran's desired appointment date is the date on which the patient or provider wants the patient to be seen. In the case of a veteran new to the system, the desired appointment date should be determined based on the veteran's preferred appointment date. See GAO, *VA Health Care: Reliability of Reported Outpatient Medical Appointment Wait Times and Scheduling Oversight Need Improvement*, GAO-13-130 (Washington, D.C.: Dec. 21, 2012).

awarded each fiscal year.[35] According to VA officials responsible for developing these performance contracts, wait times for care received from fee basis providers are excluded from these performance measures and VISN and VAMC directors' performance contracts do not include specific goals for wait times for fee basis care.

VA officials from all six VAMCs we reviewed reported that they routinely refer veterans to fee basis providers to help ensure that veterans receive timely care and that their facilities meet performance goals for wait times for VAMC-based care. For example, Biloxi VAMC officials said they refer veterans to fee basis providers to avoid having longer wait times for veterans in VAMC-based clinics that would cause the Biloxi VAMC to fall short of its performance goal for VAMC-based care wait times. Similarly, officials from the Alexandria VAMC explained that their medical center sends veterans to fee basis providers solely to meet the wait time goals for the VAMC. They said that veterans needing treatment in several specialties—including audiology, cardiology, and ophthalmology—are referred to fee basis providers to help the Alexandria VAMC meet its goals for VAMC-based clinic wait times.

While serving veterans in a timely way is important and sending them to fee basis providers may provide veterans more timely service, VA does not track how long it takes veterans to be seen by fee basis providers at all VAMCs.[36] For example, officials from the Alexandria VAMC explained that they often refer veterans to fee basis providers when the Alexandria VAMC's wait times are too long, but fee basis providers in their community also face capacity limitations and may not be able to schedule appointments for veterans any sooner than the VAMC-based provider. Since VA does not require all VAMCs to track wait times for fee basis

---

[35]Performance contracts for VISN directors are referred to as Network Director Performance Plans and performance contracts for VAMC directors are referred to as Facility Director Performance Plans. These documents include a number of performance measures with goals that VISN and VAMC directors are responsible for assuring their VISN or VAMC obtain. Performance pay for VISN and VAMC directors is determined based on their performance against these performance measures.

[36]VAMCs that have already transitioned to VA's new fee basis care administration model, referred to as Non-VA Care Coordination, are required to track the average number of days between when the VA provider entered a request for fee basis care into a veteran's medical record and the date the veteran is seen by a fee basis provider. VA set a goal for VAMCs to average 25 days or less for this to occur. However, according to VA officials, not all VAMCs are currently participating in Non-VA Care Coordination.

providers, little is known about how often veterans' wait times for fee basis care appointments exceed VAMC-based appointment wait time goals. Because VA has no data on wait times for veterans treated by fee basis providers, it is not possible to determine if veterans are receiving comparable access to fee basis providers as veterans receiving care from VAMC-based providers.[37]

VAMC Officials Reported Three Areas with the Potential to Reduce Fee Basis Spending and Utilization

Expanding VAMC Capacity

Efforts to provide either increased capacity or additional VAMC-based health care services have helped VAMCs reduce their utilization of fee basis care, according to officials from all six VAMCs we reviewed. For example, Durham VAMC officials explained that they recently completed an operating room expansion at their facility, which has allowed them to bring more surgical services back into the VAMC and reduce their reliance on fee basis surgical services. These officials also said that the Durham VAMC is preparing to expand its inpatient psychiatric unit by adding six additional inpatient beds, which will reduce their reliance on fee basis providers for treating veterans when VAMC-based psychiatric beds are at capacity. Durham VAMC officials reported that the operating room expansion saves an estimated $18 million annually and the additional six VAMC-based psychiatric unit beds saves the facility an estimated $3.4 million annually. In another case, Biloxi VAMC officials reported that in 2010 they reduced their reliance on fee basis providers for pulmonary function tests by purchasing additional equipment and hiring an additional technician to increase the VAMC-based capacity to provide these tests. As a result, officials have seen a drop in the number of veterans referred to fee basis providers for this service and fee basis costs for pulmonary function tests decreased by about $112,000 between fiscal years 2010 and 2012.

---

[37]See GAO, *Standards for Internal Control in the Federal Government*, GAO/AIMD-00-21.3.1 (Washington, D.C.: November 1999). Standards for internal control in the federal government state that agencies should design internal controls that assure ongoing monitoring occurs in the course of normal operations, is continually performed, and is ingrained in agency operations.

Such expansions require a careful analysis of the benefits and costs of the expansion. Before a VAMC expands its capacity, VA requires VAMCs to develop a business case for the expansion as part of VA's annual consideration of capital investments.[38] These business cases must address several elements—including a financial analysis and safety issues. For example, Durham VAMC officials explained that to make these decisions about expanding its operating room and inpatient psychiatric bed capacity they reviewed weekly fee basis reports that included cost and volume information on the most common services that their VAMC provided through fee basis care and used these reports to make decisions about which Durham VAMC-based services should be expanded.

However, some VAMC officials noted that it may not always be more cost effective for VAMCs to provide these services. For example, officials from the Salisbury VAMC explained that they planned to build a VAMC-based dialysis unit to reduce the number of veterans they referred to fee basis providers for dialysis treatments. However, when they compared the cost of building a dialysis unit to the cost of providing veterans dialysis treatments through fee basis providers, they determined that fee basis care was as cost-effective as building a dialysis unit.

Sharing Agreements with DOD

DOD medical facilities colocated with nearby VAMCs offer an alternative to veterans receiving care from more costly community-based fee basis providers. Currently, VA and DOD have a policy that allows the departments to charge one another at least 10 percent less for clinical

---

[38]See Department of Veterans Affairs, *Strategic Capital Investment Planning Process*, VA Handbook 0011 (Aug. 8, 2011). If a VAMC-based service expansion involves major or minor construction, VA requires VAMC officials to make a business case for the construction during VA's annual strategic capital investment process. Business cases must address a series of VA-wide criteria that address priorities such as safety, financial analysis, and client and customer access—in order to be considered for funding. VA reevaluates these criteria on a yearly basis to ensure it continually adapts to changes in demographics and health care delivery. After business cases are submitted, VA evaluates and prioritizes them for funding based on how well the suggested expansion addresses the criteria.

services than they would in locations without sharing agreements.[39] As of June 2012, there are nearly 200 active sharing agreements in place between VA and DOD that range in complexity and scope from sharing a single service to agreements that govern the sharing of multiple services.[40]

Two of the six VAMCs we reviewed—located in Las Vegas and Biloxi—share resources with neighboring DOD health care facilities to provide lower-cost care to veterans.[41] The Las Vegas VAMC has a sharing agreement with Nellis Air Force Base for some health care services, including cardiac and radiation oncology services. Similarly, the Biloxi VAMC has several sharing agreements with Air Force and Navy medical facilities along the Gulf Coast for some health care services. Officials from both these VAMCs reported that they refer veterans to these DOD facilities before sending them to fee basis providers in the community because the reimbursement rate for services provided in DOD medical facilities is lower than the Medicare rates used to reimburse fee basis providers. Officials from both the Las Vegas and Biloxi VAMCs explained that they first explore whether care is available through sharing agreements with nearby DOD medical facilities before referring the veterans to fee basis providers.

---

[39]In fiscal year 2003, a memorandum of understanding between VA and DOD established a policy for reimbursement for health care services that they share. This memorandum of understanding allows VA and DOD collaborating facilities to use at least a 10 percent discount from the standard allowable charge for clinical services and certain specialty services. VA uses the fee basis care claims process to reimburse DOD medical facilities for the care they provide veterans through sharing agreements. DOD is reimbursed for services provided to veterans using the same process as fee basis providers, but their services are reimbursed at rates specified in each individual sharing agreement.

[40]For more information, see GAO, *VA and DOD Health Care: Department-Level Actions Needed to Assess Collaboration Performance, Address Barriers, and Identify Opportunities,* GAO-12-992 (Washington, D.C.: Sept. 28, 2012). In September 2012, we recommended that the Secretaries of Veterans Affairs and Defense further develop a systematic process for identifying and furthering collaboration opportunities, such as sharing agreements. Both VA and DOD generally concurred with this recommendation but stressed the importance of local leaders in the development of collaboration because these local officials have the best sense of their health care markets.

[41]Both the Las Vegas and Biloxi VAMCs participate in 2 of 10 joint ventures with DOD facilities in place throughout the country. Joint ventures allow VA and DOD to share multiple health care services and sometimes share facilities and give VA and DOD increased flexibility to determine reimbursement rates than with sharing agreements alone.

Transferring Veterans Back to VAMC-based Inpatient Care

Another critical factor affecting fee basis care spending and utilization is the timely transfer of veterans receiving inpatient care from fee basis providers back to VAMC-based care. This is particularly relevant because, as we discussed earlier, VA has spent almost $1.3 billion over the last 5 years on emergency inpatient services for veterans through the Millennium Act and about $4.6 billion on preauthorized inpatient fee basis care. (See app. II.) As a result, it is important that VAMC staff closely monitor the conditions of veterans receiving inpatient care from fee basis providers to ensure that they are transferred to VAMCs once their conditions stabilize. Officials from all six VAMCs we examined reported that transferring veterans being treated by fee basis providers back to VAMC-based care when appropriate can be a way of reducing the cost of inpatient fee basis care. According to officials at two VAMCs, this is because VAMC inpatient bed capacity limitations that required a veteran to be referred to an inpatient fee basis provider can change during the course of a veteran's hospital stay in non-VA facilities.

While officials from all six VAMCs we reviewed noted that transferring veterans back to inpatient VAMC-based care can help reduce fee basis utilization and spending, we found some VAMCs have more robust monitoring methods than other VAMCs for tracking veterans being treated by fee basis providers through their utilization management programs.[42] Specifically, we found the following:

- Three of the VAMCs we reviewed had a more formal approach that was integrated with their utilization management programs to actively identify circumstances when veterans being treated as inpatients by fee basis providers could return to the VAMC to complete their inpatient care. For example, the Salisbury VAMC has a transfer coordinator program specifically designated to actively identify such circumstances. The Salisbury VAMC employs a nurse case manager who visits veterans during their inpatient stays with fee basis

---

[42]See Veterans Health Administration, *Utilization Management Program*, VHA Directive 2010-021 (May 14, 2010). VA policy requires that all VAMCs have a utilization management program in place. These programs are a key tool for managing the daily inpatient flow of a VAMC and ensuring that veterans receiving care at the VAMC are receiving the appropriate services based on their clinical needs; that information is gathered to inform decision making related to patient care management and discharge coordination; and that delays in services are identified. Utilization management often results in improved operational efficiencies, such as decreased lengths-of-stay at the VAMC and enhanced access for veterans.

providers and identifies changes in veterans' conditions that will allow them to return to the VAMC, and coordinates veterans' transitions back into VAMC-based care. According to Salisbury VAMC officials, this program has allowed them to transfer veterans back to the VAMC to complete their care once the veterans' conditions have stabilized.

- In contrast, the other three VAMCs we reviewed had a more passive approach that was limited to tracking veterans' progress through information given to them by the veterans' inpatient fee basis providers. For example, the Alexandria VAMC's transfer coordinator monitors veterans' inpatient fee basis care; however, this information is rarely used to transfer veterans back to the VAMC to complete their treatment.

Although ensuring that VAMCs are incorporating fee basis care into their utilization management programs would enable VA to more efficiently identify when opportunities exist for some veterans to be transferred back to lower-cost VAMC-based care, VA does not currently require all VAMCs to conduct such review.[43] Specifically, VA's current utilization management policy does not require VAMCs to incorporate reviews of inpatient fee basis care into their VAMC-based utilization management programs.[44] VA Central Office has not provided guidance to all VAMCs on how to most effectively track veterans receiving inpatient care from fee basis providers, which has allowed VAMC programs to take a variety of forms. Ultimately, without guidance and standardized procedures provided by VA Central Office, some VAMCs may not be monitoring veterans receiving inpatient care from fee basis providers in the

---

[43]VAMCs that have already transitioned to VA's new fee basis care administration model, referred to as Non-VA Care Coordination, have processes in place to coordinate with non-VA facilities and gather information needed to determine if transferring veterans back to the VAMC for continued treatment is possible and place this information in the fee basis care coordination system and veterans' medical records. These processes include documenting VA bed availability, the medical necessity of the treatment veterans are receiving in a non-VA facility, and when the veteran is stable enough for transfer. However, these VAMCs follow local transfer procedures to determine whether or not veterans receiving care from inpatient fee basis providers in the community will be transferred back to the VAMC and not all VAMCs are currently participating in Non-VA Care Coordination.

[44]See GAO/AIMD-00-21.3.1. Standards for internal control in the federal government state that management and employees should establish and maintain an environment throughout the organization that sets a positive and supportive attitude toward internal control and conscientious management.

community closely enough to prevent prolonged and unnecessary stays for veterans in inpatient fee basis care and may be missing other opportunities to reduce fee basis care spending.

VA's Processes for Overseeing the Fee Basis Care Program Lack Critical Data Needed to Effectively Track and Monitor Fee Basis Spending and Utilization

One of VHA CBO's three primary methods for monitoring fee basis care spending and utilization is its review of fee basis data. According to VHA CBO officials, these reviews are primarily focused on examining fee basis care utilization and spending—including VISN fee basis care utilization and significant high-cost areas, such as dialysis treatment. Analysis of fee basis data is an important aspect of monitoring that allows VHA CBO staff to look for outliers in spending and utilization, mistakes in fee basis claims data, potential lost opportunities to reduce spending and utilization, and to assess more long-term considerations—such as adjusting the level of fee basis care services or assessing potential areas for VAMC-based service expansion. However, the usefulness of this monitoring method as an oversight tool is significantly limited due to the way fee basis data are collected and reported to the VHA CBO.

Currently, VA's data system collects claims data for each individual service provided by a fee basis provider—such as the physician's time, surgical procedures, hospital rooms, and laboratory tests—rather than the total cost of a veteran's office visit or inpatient stay. VA's current data system cannot group these individual services by episode of care—a combined total of all care provided to a veteran during a single office visit or inpatient stay.[45,46] For example, during an office visit to an orthopedic surgeon for a joint replacement evaluation, an X-ray for the affected joint may be ordered, the veteran may be given a blood test, and the veteran may receive a physical evaluation from the orthopedic surgeon. The fee basis provider would submit a bill to VA for the office visit and separate bills would be submitted by the radiologist that X-rayed the affected joint

---

[45] See GAO, *Medicare: Private Sector Initiatives to Bundle Hospital and Physician Payments for an Episode of Care*, GAO-11-126R (Washington, D.C.: Jan. 31, 2011).

[46] In March 2013, VHA CBO officials told us that for inpatient claims they could construct a program to group inpatient and inpatient ancillary claims together by linking all the records of individual services provided to veterans during a particular date range. However, this method relies on correct local VISN and VAMC data entry into VA's fee basis data system and correct information to be provided by providers. VHA CBO officials acknowledged that there is no way to link outpatient services together to create a record of a single outpatient episode of care.

and the lab that performed the veteran's blood test. Each of these bills would include charges under different medical billing codes.[47] The VISN or VAMC-based fee basis clerk processing this claim would record these charges in VA's basis claims processing software and request payment for these fee basis providers. However, the fee basis data system used by VHA CBO to review these payments would not be able to link the charges for these three treatments together as a single episode of care for this veteran's office visit with an orthopedic surgeon.

Not being able to group charges from fee basis providers by episode of care has the following disadvantages in terms of monitoring fee basis care and potentially reducing costs:

- **Monitoring challenges**. From a monitoring perspective, not having data by episode of care prevents VA from efficiently identifying areas of utilization growth or unusually high spending. For example, VA-wide episode of care monitoring would allow VHA CBO to assess whether opportunities for strategic expansion of VAMC-based services—such as the Durham VAMC operating room expansion and the Biloxi VAMC addition of pulmonary function test equipment mentioned earlier—would be possible in more VAMCs. Episode of care monitoring would more effectively allow VA to make more consistent strategic decisions about such service expansions.

- **Cost analysis limitations**. From a cost perspective, not having fee basis data on an episode of care basis prevents VA from efficiently assessing whether fee basis providers were reimbursed appropriately. Without the ability to monitor fee basis spending by episodes of care, VHA CBO cannot conduct retrospective reviews of VISN and VAMC claims to determine if the appropriate rate was applied for the care provided by fee basis providers. For example, VHA CBO staff cannot verify that fee basis care that should be paid using Medicare

---

[47]Fee basis providers bill for their services using individual Healthcare Common Procedure Coding System (HCPCS) codes or Medicare-Severity Diagnosis-Related Group (MS-DRG) codes, which are the standard medical billing codes for outpatient and inpatient medical care, to account for various treatments that are provided during the same office or clinic visit or inpatient stay. HCPCS is a collection of standardized codes that represent medical procedures, supplies, products, and services. The system contains two types of codes—level I codes (also referred to as current procedural terminology codes) that consist of five numeric digits, and level II codes that consist of a letter followed by four numeric digits. MS-DRG codes classify inpatient stays according to both patients' clinical conditions and the services patients receive.

"bundled" reimbursement rates were in fact paid using these bundled rates because all individual charges from a veteran's episode of care cannot be reliably linked. Since VA uses Medicare rates to reimburse fee basis providers for most services, VAMCs and VISNs, like Medicare, use bundled reimbursement rates for some procedures that provide a single payment for closely related services in some cases. Bundled rates are designed to give providers an incentive to furnish care more efficiently as providers retain the difference if the bundled payment exceeds the cost of care.[48] Bundled rates provide a financial incentive for delivering care more efficiently by making providers accountable if a patient's treatment costs exceeded the bundled rate.

To effectively conduct these retrospective reviews, VHA CBO would need to change its claims processing methods and ensure that the VISN or VAMC fee basis clerks processing each provider's claims assign a claim number to each payment made to a fee basis provider for an episode of care. This claim number would serve as a linkage among the individual service line items in VA's fee basis data system and allow VHA CBO to group together all payments made for a single episode of care and assess the total cost of that episode of care.[49]

---

[48] See GAO-11-126R.

[49] VHA CBO staff use data extracted from the fee basis claims processing software and other databases to monitor the fee basis care program. The fee basis claims processing software includes many data fields that are not transferred to VHA CBO for analysis. In September 2012, VHA CBO fee basis data management officials reported that VA plans to incorporate a claim number into its fee basis claims processing software package used by VISN and VAMC-based fee basis claims processing clerks to review and authorize payments to fee basis providers. Without ensuring VHA CBO staff have access to this claim number, these officials said they will not be able to analyze and track fee basis care spending and utilization by episodes of care.

VA Is Currently Implementing a Short-Term Corrective Action Plan for the Fee Basis Care Program, but Longer-Term Strategy Is Still in Development

In September 2012, VA outlined both short- and long-term plans for improving the fee basis care program following problems highlighted by several OIG audits and a recent congressional hearing. The short-term corrective action plan is made up of a series of tasks to be completed in fiscal year 2013 across six key areas—(1) foundational activities, (2) achieving a sustainable decrease in fee basis care improper payments, (3) recovery and recapture of fee basis care overpayments, (4) building a culture of accountability within the fee basis care program, (5) enhancing internal controls and data integrity, and (6) training and educating VISNs and VAMCs.

We found that VA has taken a number of steps to better ensure the completion of its short-term corrective action plan in fiscal year 2013.[50] Specifically, VA has identified clear leadership for tasks, created teams to accomplish tasks that include representatives from across VA operations, sought the input of internal stakeholders—such as VISN and VAMC fee basis unit staff—and external stakeholders—including the VA OIG, set clear target dates for the completion of tasks, and identified methods for assessing whether or not tasks had the desired effect on the fee basis care program. While it is still too early to determine if the efforts included in the short-term corrective action plan will produce meaningful improvements in the fee basis care program, it represents an important first step in increasing accountability for the outcomes of the fee basis care program. (See table 1.)

---

[50]GAO, *Executive Guide: Effectively Implementing the Government Performance and Results Act*, GAO/GGD-96-118 (Washington, D.C.: June 1996). When other leading public-sector organizations are engaged in efforts to improve their performance and help their organizations become more effective—similar to VA's goals for the short-term corrective action plan—we found that these organizations commonly take three steps: (1) define a clear mission and goals, (2) measure performance to gauge progress toward achieving goals, and (3) use performance information as a basis for decision making.

Table 1: Status of Short-Term Improvement Goals, March 2013

Short-term improvement goals	Estimated completion date	Completion progress
Foundational activities		
• Complete realignment of regulations to applicable statutes and revise applicable handbooks and directives	December 2013	◐
• Implement a national contracting strategy	June 2013	◐
Achieve a sustainable decrease in improper payments		
• Implement new care coordination initiative	September 2013	◐
• Implement cost estimation process improvements	March 2013	◐
• Evaluate the effectiveness of fee basis provider outreach efforts	September 2013	◐
• Validate the effectiveness of new Medicare-based fee schedule and software updates to help fee basis claims processing clerks identify the appropriate payment rate for claims	March 2013	●
Recover and recapture overpayments		
• Initiate recapture activities as appropriate with a former contract service provider found to overpay fee basis providers	March 2013	◐
• Assess recapture management approach and create a stronger partnership with VISN and VAMC Chief Financial Officers	June 2013	◐
Build a culture of accountability		
• Initiate communication with senior leaders—including VA Central Office officials, VISN leadership, and VAMC-based fee basis unit managers	December 2012	●
• Define roles and responsibilities for the fee basis care program	June 2013	◐
Enhance internal controls and data integrity		
• Visit the 30 lowest-performing fee basis care units and develop action plans for improvement	September 2013	◐
• Assess fee basis care web-based performance management tools and ensure these tools provide a clear picture of the program's performance	March 2013	◐
• Increase communication to VISN and VAMC fee basis care units	December 2012	●
• Implement predictive auditing to provide near-real time projections of fee basis care improper payments	March 2013	◐
Train and educate the field		
• Create a high performing education initiative that promotes learning and training on improper payment risks and control issues	March 2013	◐
• Mandate appropriate training courses	No date specified[a]	◐
• Update fee basis training courses to reflect the content of a new competency model developed for fee basis staff	September 2013	◐

Key: ● = completed; ◐ = in progress

Source: GAO.

[a] In February 2013, VHA CBO informed us that these training mandates are currently being discussed with VA's labor relations partners and they did not have an estimated completion date for these discussions.

VA is also in the process of developing a long-term strategy for improving its fee basis care program. This long-term strategy includes efforts to develop and implement a new organizational structure for the fee basis care program, consolidate claims processing functions in fewer locations, develop comprehensive guidance for the fee basis care program, implement a new competency-based personnel model, and implement new claims processing software efforts. To date, progress on the development of this long-term strategy has been limited to the development of new claims processing software and initial discussions of the new organizational structure. In February 2013, VA officials told us that the long-term strategy is still in development.

Conclusions

VA's fee basis care program is a critical means for providing accessible health care to veterans. VA has acknowledged that fee basis care is a necessary tool for veterans when a VAMC does not have an available clinical specialist or when veterans face long travel distances to obtain care from VAMC-based providers. VA has also made concerted efforts in recent years to improve the fee basis care program by implementing a number of initiatives designed to improve the program—including new software packages for VISN and VAMC fee basis claims processing units, a new care coordination program, and initiating a program to better coordinate with fee basis providers.

Moving forward, we believe it is critical that VA address four areas as potential ways to more effectively manage and monitor the fee basis care program. First, veterans' eligibility for travel reimbursement may affect whether they are referred to fee basis care or to another VAMC. Some veterans who qualify for travel reimbursement under VA's beneficiary travel program might elect to seek care at another VAMC without incurring personal travel expenses in lieu of being treated by a fee basis provider. In some cases, this could result in VA paying less for their care than it would if the veteran were treated through the fee basis care program. Should the Secretary of Veterans Affairs exercise his ability to revise the beneficiary travel eligibility requirements to allow for the use of beneficiary travel in cases where it is both more cost-effective for VA and in the veteran's best interest to receive care at another VAMC instead of a fee basis provider, it could be possible to lower overall fee basis care utilization and spending. In addition, VA does not currently require VAMCs to assess either the cost-effectiveness of reimbursing veterans for travel to another VAMC when determining whether to preauthorize fee basis care in veterans' local communities.

Second, VA should better manage fee basis care wait times and costs. VA currently does not include fee basis care wait times in the measures it uses to assess VISN and VAMC directors' performance and does not track the amount of time veterans wait to see a fee basis provider. As a result, the VAMCs we reviewed are referring veterans to fee basis providers to ensure they meet the wait time performance goals for VAMC-based clinics. Having data on wait times for veterans referred to fee basis providers would help VA better determine if veterans are receiving comparable access to fee basis providers and VAMC-based providers.

Third, VA may be missing an opportunity to reduce the cost of inpatient fee basis care by not requiring VAMC-based utilization management programs designed to regularly assess VAMC capacity to consider veterans being treated by non-VA inpatient fee basis providers. Incorporating veterans treated by non-VA inpatient fee basis providers into ongoing VAMC utilization management programs would allow VAMCs to identify situations when they no longer have capacity limitations and can complete a veteran's treatment in-house at a lower cost than the fee basis provider.

Finally, VA can also improve its capability to more effectively monitor the fee basis care program. VA Central Office's monitoring efforts are limited by the inability to analyze fee basis care data by episode of care. Because information that would allow VA to pull together all services with a single office visit or inpatient stay is not available, VA Central Office cannot effectively monitor the payments made by fee basis care units or ensure that fee basis providers are billing VA appropriately for care.

Recommendations for Executive Action

To effectively manage fee basis care spending, we recommend that the Secretary of Veterans Affairs take the following action:

- Revise the beneficiary travel eligibility regulations to allow for the reimbursement of travel expenses for veterans to another VAMC to receive needed medical care when it is more cost-effective and appropriate for the veteran than seeking similar care from a fee basis provider.

To effectively manage fee basis care wait times and spending, we recommend that the Secretary of Veterans Affairs direct the Under Secretary for Health to take the following three actions:

- Require during the fee basis authorization process that VA providers and fee basis officials determine the cost-effectiveness of reimbursing medically stable veterans eligible for beneficiary travel for travel to another VAMC rather than referring them to a fee basis provider for similar care.

- Analyze the amount of time veterans wait to see fee basis providers and apply the same wait time goals to fee basis care that are used as VAMC-based wait time performance measures.

- Establish guidance for VAMCs that specifies how fee basis care should be incorporated with other VAMC utilization management efforts.

To ensure that VA Central Office effectively monitors fee basis care, we recommend that the Secretary of Veterans Affairs direct the Under Secretary for Health to take the following action:

- Ensure that fee basis data include a claim number that will allow for VA Central Office to analyze the episode of care costs for fee basis care.

Agency Comments and Our Evaluation

VA provided written comments on a draft of this report, which we have reprinted in appendix III. In its comments, VA generally agreed with our conclusions, concurred with our five recommendations, and described the agency's plans to implement each of our recommendations. VA also provided technical comments, which we have incorporated as appropriate.

In its plan, VA stated that to address our first recommendation, VHA CBO will consider including provisions related to veterans' travel reimbursement to another VAMC to receive needed medical care when it is more cost-effective and appropriate during a planned upcoming revision to the agency's beneficiary travel regulations.

To address our second recommendation, VA noted that it is working to revise procedures for both its new fee basis care administration model, referred to as Non-VA Care Coordination, and the beneficiary travel program to ensure that the cost-effectiveness of a veterans' travel to another VAMC or to a non-VA care provider is reviewed as part of the authorization of fee basis care and is included in standard operating procedures and training.

To address our third recommendation, VA noted that VHA CBO is completing requirements for a national consolidated monthly wait time indicator to measure performance for fee basis care referrals. However, VA did not acknowledge whether or not the wait time indicators used in this monthly indicator would be the same as those used for VAMC-based care, as we recommended. We support VA's decision to set wait time goals for fee basis care, but we believe the agency should ensure that wait time goals used for fee basis care are the same as those applied to VAMC-based care.

To address our fourth recommendation, VA stated that the new fee basis care administration model, Non-VA Care Coordination, includes a template for managing information transfers from non-VA providers to VA staff that will support the utilization management practices of VAMCs. We support VA's efforts to standardize this information exchange in its fee basis care administration practices, but encourage the agency to also clarify its utilization management policies to ensure that VAMC utilization management staff regularly coordinate with VAMC fee basis management staff to receive this information from non-VA providers.

Finally, to address our fifth recommendation, VA noted that the agency agrees that analyzing episode of care costs is an important part of the agency's fee basis monitoring activities. VA outlined its plan to analyze existing data systems and determine the most cost-effective method for monitoring episode of care costs.

We are sending copies of this report to the Secretary of Veterans Affairs, the Under Secretary for Health, appropriate congressional committees, and other interested parties. In addition, the report is available at no charge on the GAO website at http://www.gao.gov.

If you or your staffs have any questions about this report, please contact me at (202) 512-7114 or at williamsonr@gao.gov. Contact points for our Offices of Congressional Relations and Public Affairs may be found on the last page of this report. GAO staff who made major contributions to this report are listed in appendix IV.

Randall B. Williamson
Director, Health Care

List of Requesters

The Honorable Patty Murray
Chairman
Committee on the Budget
United States Senate

The Honorable Bernie Sanders
Chairman
The Honorable Richard Burr
Ranking Member
Committee on Veterans' Affairs
United States Senate

The Honorable Jeff Miller
Chairman
The Honorable Michael Michaud
Ranking Member
Committee on Veterans' Affairs
House of Representatives

The Honorable Mike Coffman
Chairman
Subcommittee on Oversight and Investigations
Committee on Veterans' Affairs
House of Representatives

The Honorable Bill Johnson
House of Representatives

Appendix I: VA Spending and Utilization by Fee Basis Care Category

This appendix provides additional results from our analysis of Department of Veterans Affairs (VA) fee basis data from fiscal years 2008 through 2012. Specifically, the table below provides additional information on how much VA spent on fee basis care and how many unique veterans received care from fee basis providers by fee basis care categories.

Table: VA Spending and Utilization by Fee Basis Care Category, Fiscal Years 2008 through 2012

VA fee basis care category	Spending dollars in billions[a]	Percentage of total fee basis spending	Utilization number of unique veterans[b]	Percentage of total fee basis utilization[c]
Preauthorized outpatient	7.36	36.28	1,871,984	76.50
Preauthorized inpatient	4.60	22.68	268,763	10.98
Home health	2.69	13.28	327,514	13.38
Community nursing home	2.50	12.33	63,714	2.60
Millennium Act[d]	1.79	8.83	373,738	15.27
Emergency care for veterans with service-connected conditions[e]	0.91	4.50	161,359	6.59
Dental	0.36	1.77	151,419	6.19
Compensation and pension exams	0.07	0.33	142,212	5.81

Source: GAO (analysis); VA (data).

Notes: Fee basis spending and utilization in this table does not include pharmacy-only fee basis care. Pharmacy-only fee basis care consists of reimbursements to veterans for medications that they paid for as part of emergency care that was reimbursed by VA under 38 U.S.C. § 1728 (emergency care generally for service-connected conditions) or 38 U.S.C. § 1725 (Veterans Millennium Health Care and Benefits Act emergency care for non-service-connected conditions). Total spending for pharmacy-only fee basis care was $0.002 billion for fiscal years 2008 through 2012. A total of 11,750 unique veterans received such reimbursement from fiscal year 2008 through fiscal year 2012.

[a]Spending amounts may not sum to spending totals cited previously in text due to rounding.

[b]Utilization amounts may not match utilization totals cited previously in text, as veterans may have received care in multiple categories during fiscal years 2008 through 2012. To determine the fee basis utilization numbers in this table, we counted each individual veteran once per fee basis care category by identifying the number of unique Social Security numbers present in fee basis data for fiscal years 2008 through 2012.

[c]Utilization percentages may not add to 100 percent due to rounding and because some veterans may have received fee basis care in multiple categories.

[d]Millennium Act care refers to services provided to veterans under the 1999 Veterans Millennium Health Care and Benefits Act. Under this act, VA is authorized to pay emergency care costs for some veterans' non-service-connected conditions, among other things. See 38 U.S.C. § 1725.

[e]Emergency care for veterans with service-connected conditions refers to fee basis care that meets the eligibility requirements for emergency care under 38 U.S.C. § 1728. Under this statute, VA is required to pay for emergency care provided by non-VA facilities for service-connected conditions, non-service-connected conditions associated with and aggravating a service-connected condition, any condition if the veteran is classified by VA as permanently and totally disabled from a service-connected condition, and any condition for veterans participating in a vocational rehabilitation program who need care to participate in a course of training.

Appendix II: VA Outpatient and Inpatient Spending and Utilization by Fee Basis Care Category

This appendix provides additional results from our analysis of Department of Veterans Affairs (VA) fee basis data from fiscal years 2008 through 2012.

- Table 3 provides additional information on how much VA spent on outpatient fee basis care and how many unique veterans received care from outpatient fee basis providers by fee basis care categories.

- Table 4 provides additional information on how much VA spent on inpatient fee basis care and how many unique veterans received care from inpatient fee basis providers by fee basis care categories.

Table 3: Outpatient Spending and Utilization by VA Fee Basis Care Category, Fiscal Years 2008 through 2012

VA fee basis care category	Outpatient spending (dollars in billions)	Percentage of total outpatient spending[a]	Outpatient utilization (number of unique veterans)[b]	Percentage of total outpatient utilization[c]
Preauthorized	7.36	65.59	1,871,984	79.57
Home health	2.69	24.01	327,514	13.92
Millennium Act[d]	0.49	4.41	311,199	13.23
Dental	0.36	3.20	151,419	6.44
Emergency care for veterans with service-connected conditions[e]	0.25	2.20	126,896	5.39
Compensation and pension exams	0.07	0.60	142,212	6.04

Source: GAO (analysis); VA (data).

Notes: Fee basis spending and utilization in this table does not include pharmacy-only fee basis care. Pharmacy-only fee basis care consists of reimbursements to veterans for medications that they paid for as part of emergency care that was reimbursed by VA under 38 U.S.C. § 1728 (emergency care generally for service-connected conditions) or 38 U.S.C. § 1725 (Veterans Millennium Health Care and Benefits Act emergency care for non-service-connected conditions). Total spending for pharmacy-only fee basis care was $0.002 billion for fiscal years 2008 through 2012. A total of 11,750 unique veterans received such reimbursement from fiscal year 2008 through fiscal year 2012.

[a]Spending percentages may not sum to 100 percent due to rounding.

[b]Utilization amounts may not match utilization totals cited previously in text, as veterans may have received care in multiple categories during fiscal years 2008 through 2012. To determine the fee basis utilization numbers in this table, we counted each individual veteran once per fee basis care category by identifying the number of unique Social Security numbers present in outpatient fee basis data for fiscal years 2008 through 2012.

[c]Utilization percentages may not add to 100 percent due to rounding and because some veterans may have received fee basis care in multiple categories.

[d]Millennium Act care refers to services provided to veterans under the 1999 Veterans Millennium Health Care and Benefits Act. Under this act, VA is authorized to pay emergency care costs for some veterans' non-service-connected conditions, among other things. See 38 U.S.C. § 1725.

[e]Emergency care for veterans with service-connected conditions refers to fee basis care that meets the eligibility requirements for emergency care under 38 U.S.C. § 1728. Under this statute, VA is required to pay for emergency care provided by non-VA facilities for service-connected conditions, non-service-connected conditions associated with and aggravating a service-connected condition, any condition if the veteran is classified by VA as permanently and totally disabled from a service-

Appendix II: VA Outpatient Patient Spending and Utilization by Fee Basis Care Category

connected condition, and any condition for veterans participating in a vocational rehabilitation program who need care to participate in a course of training.

Table 4: Patient Spending and Utilization by VA Fee Basis Care Category, Fiscal Years 2008 through 2012

VA Fee Basis Care Category	Patient spending dollars in billions	Percentage of total patient spending	Patient utilization number of unique veterans[a]	Percentage of total patient utilization[b]
Preauthorized	4.60	50.76	268,763	56.96
Community nursing home	2.50	27.58	63,714	13.50
Millennium Act[c]	1.30	14.30	163,647	34.68
Emergency care for veterans with service-connected conditions[d]	0.67	7.36	65,309	13.84

Source: GAO (analysis); VA (data).

Notes: Fee basis spending and utilization in this table does not include pharmacy-only fee basis care. Pharmacy-only fee basis care consists of reimbursements to veterans for medications that they paid for as part of emergency care that was reimbursed by VA under 38 U.S.C. § 1728 (emergency care generally for service-connected conditions) or 38 U.S.C. § 1725 (Veterans Millennium Health Care and Benefits Act emergency care for non-service-connected conditions). Total spending for pharmacy-only fee basis care was $0.002 billion for fiscal years 2008 through 2012. A total of 11,750 unique veterans received such reimbursement from fiscal year 2008 through fiscal year 2012.

[a]Utilization amounts may not match utilization totals cited previously in text, as veterans may have received care in multiple categories during fiscal years 2008 through 2012. To determine the fee basis utilization numbers in this table, we counted each individual veteran once per fee basis care category by identifying the number of unique Social Security numbers present in inpatient fee basis data for fiscal years 2008 through 2012.

[b]Utilization percentages may not add to 100 percent due to rounding and because some veterans may have received fee basis care in multiple categories.

[c]Millennium Act care refers to services provided to veterans under the 1999 Veterans Millennium Health Care and Benefits Act. Under this act, VA is authorized to pay emergency care costs for some veterans' non-service-connected conditions, among other things. See 38 U.S.C. § 1725.

[d]Emergency care for veterans with service-connected conditions refers to fee basis care that meets the eligibility requirements for emergency care under 38 U.S.C. § 1728. Under this statute, VA is required to pay for emergency care provided by non-VA facilities for service-connected conditions, non-service-connected conditions associated with and aggravating a service-connected condition, any condition if the veteran is classified by VA as permanently and totally disabled from a service-connected condition, and any condition for veterans participating in a vocational rehabilitation program who need care to participate in a course of training.

Appendix III: Comments from the Department of Veterans Affairs

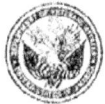

DEPARTMENT OF VETERANS AFFAIRS
Washington DC 20420

May 16, 2013

Mr. Randall Williamson
Director, Health Care
U.S. Government Accountability Office
441 G Street, NW
Washington, DC 20548

Dear Mr. Williamson:

The Department of Veterans Affairs (VA) has reviewed the Government Accountability Office's (GAO) draft report, *"VA HEALTH CARE: Management and Oversight of Fee Basis Care Need Improvement"* (GAO-13-441) and generally agrees with GAO's conclusions and concurs with GAO's five recommendations to the Department.

The enclosure specifically addresses GAO's five recommendations and provides an action plan for each. VA appreciates the opportunity to comment on your draft report.

Sincerely,

Jose D. Riojas
Interim Chief of Staff

Enclosure

Appendix I: Comments from the Department
of Veterans Affairs

Enclosure

Department of Veterans Affairs (VA) Comments to
Government Accountability Office (GAO) Draft Report
*"VA HEALTH CARE: Management and Oversight of Fee
Basis Care Need Improvement"*
(GAO-13-441)

GAO Recommendation: To effectively manage fee basis care spending, we recommend that the Secretary of Veterans Affairs take the following action:

Recommendation 1: Revise the beneficiary travel eligibility regulations to allow for the reimbursement of travel expenses for veterans to another VAMC to receive needed medical care when it is more cost-effective and appropriate for the veteran than seeking similar care from a fee basis provider.

VA Comment: Concur. The Veterans Health Administration's (VHA) Chief Business Office (CBO) will consider including provisions related to reimbursement of travel expenses for Veterans to another VA medical center (VAMC) to receive needed medical care when it is more cost-effective and appropriate in conjunction with the planned revision of VA's beneficiary travel regulations. Relevant decision making will take into account Veteran's choice as to place of care; medical condition(s); ability to travel; required family support; and other relevant circumstances.

GAO Recommendation: To effectively manage fee basis care wait times and spending, we recommend that the Secretary of Veterans Affairs direct the Under Secretary for Health to take the following three actions:

Recommendation 2: Require during the fee basis authorization process that VA providers and fee basis officials determine the cost-effectiveness of reimbursing medically stable veterans eligible for beneficiary travel for travel to another VAMC rather than referring them to a fee basis provider for similar care.

VA Comment: Concur. VHA's Non-VA Care Coordination (NVCC)[1] and Beneficiary Travel teams are working together to revise procedures and ensure that the cost-effectiveness of a Veteran's travel to another VAMC or to a non-VA care provider is reviewed as part of the NVCC consult/authorization activity, and is part of standard operating procedures and training.

Recommendation 3: Analyze the amount of time veterans wait to see fee basis providers and apply the same wait time goals to fee basis care that are used as VAMC-based wait time performance measures.

VA Comment: Concur. VHA's CBO is completing requirements for building a national-level, consolidated monthly wait time indicator report for measuring performance for non-VA medical care purchases. Anticipated completion date: September 30, 2013

---

[1] Non-VA Care Coordination (NVCC) is a nationwide effort to improve and standardize non-VA care (Fee Basis) coordination processes across VHA.

Enclosure

Department of Veterans Affairs (VA) Comments to
Government Accountability Office (GAO) Draft Report
*"VA HEALTH CARE: Management and Oversight of Fee
Basis Care Need Improvement"*
(GAO-13-441)

Recommendation 4: Establish guidance for VAMCs that specifies how fee basis care should be incorporated with other VAMC utilization management efforts.

VA Comment: Concur. VHA's CBO is in the process of fully implementing NVCC. Once NVCC is fully implemented, the utilization of standardized template progress notes titled "Non-VA Care Hospital Notification" and "Non-VA Care Coordination Note" will support utilization management practices. Anticipated completion date: September 30, 2013

GAO Recommendation: To ensure that VA Central Office effectively monitors fee basis care, we recommend that the Secretary of Veterans Affairs direct the Under Secretary for Health to take the following action:

Recommendation 5: Ensure that fee basis data include a claim number that will allow VA Central Office to analyze the episode of care costs for fee basis care.

VA Comment: Concur. VHA concurs with analyzing episodes of care cost, however, incorporating the claim number in Fee Basis Claim System (FBCS) is not the best long-term solution for gathering episode of care cost data. To address the issue of analyzing episode of care cost, CBO is taking the following actions:

CBO is in the process of completing the analysis of data from the Corporate Data Warehouse and Program Integrity Tool that will allow for analysis of episode of care costs. Upon completion of the analysis, VA will decide the most cost effective method for monitoring episodes of care costs. Anticipated completion date: August 1, 2013

- CBO plans to implement the Healthcare Claims Processing (HCP) system, which will also allow for episodes of care cost analysis. HCP is VHA's future state claims processing system and it is currently under development. VHA-wide implementation will take approximately 9 months to a year and is expected to start around December of 2014. Anticipated completion date: October 1, 2015

- Since the GAO audit, Patch 22 (Program Integrity Tool) in the FBCS has been implemented. The patch now provides a method of integrating, sending and receiving, tracking and managing claims so that analysis of the episode of care costs can be completed for claims that are processed through FBCS. Patch 22 also assigns a unique claim key number (similar to a claim number) to all claims associated with an episode of care within the FBCS. This unique claim key number can be used to monitor episode of care costs.

Appendix IV: GAO Contact and Staff Acknowledgments

GAO Contact	Randall B. Williamson, (202) 512-7114 or williamsonr@gao.gov
Staff Acknowledgments	In addition to the contact named above, Marcia A. Mann, Assistant Director; Kathleen Diamond; Krister Friday; Katherine Nicole Laubacher; Daniel K. Lee; Lisa Motley; Rebecca Rust Williamson; and Malissa G. Winograd made key contributions to this report.

GAO's Mission	The Government Accountability Office, the audit, evaluation, and investigative arm of Congress, exists to support Congress in meeting its constitutional responsibilities and to help improve the performance and accountability of the federal government for the American people. GAO examines the use of public funds; evaluates federal programs and policies; and provides analyses, recommendations, and other assistance to help Congress make informed oversight, policy, and funding decisions. GAO's commitment to good government is reflected in its core values of accountability, integrity, and reliability.
Obtaining Copies of GAO Reports and Testimony	The fastest and easiest way to obtain copies of GAO documents at no cost is through GAO's website (http://www.gao.gov). Each weekday afternoon, GAO posts on its website newly released reports, testimony, and correspondence. To have GAO e-mail you a list of newly posted products, go to http://www.gao.gov and select "E-mail Updates."
Order by Phone	The price of each GAO publication reflects GAO's actual cost of production and distribution and depends on the number of pages in the publication and whether the publication is printed in color or black and white. Pricing and ordering information is posted on GAO's website, http://www.gao.gov/ordering.htm. Place orders by calling (202) 512-6000, toll free (866) 801-7077, or TDD (202) 512-2537. Orders may be paid for using American Express, Discover Card, MasterCard, Visa, check, or money order. Call for additional information.
Connect with GAO	Connect with GAO on Facebook, Flickr, Twitter, and YouTube. Subscribe to our RSS Feeds or E-mail Updates. Listen to our Podcasts. Visit GAO on the web at www.gao.gov.
To Report Fraud, Waste, and Abuse in Federal Programs	Contact: Website: http://www.gao.gov/fraudnet/fraudnet.htm E-mail: fraudnet@gao.gov Automated answering system: (800) 424-5454 or (202) 512-7470
Congressional Relations	Katherine Siggerud, Managing Director, siggerudk@gao.gov, (202) 512-4400, U.S. Government Accountability Office, 441 G Street NW, Room 7125, Washington, DC 20548
Public Affairs	Chuck Young, Managing Director, youngc1@gao.gov, (202) 512-4800 U.S. Government Accountability Office, 441 G Street NW, Room 7149 Washington, DC 20548

Please Print on Recycled Paper.

www.ingramcontent.com/pod-product-compliance
Lightning Source LLC
Chambersburg PA
CBHW081910170526
45167CB00007B/3222